CHAPTER 1

MY LIFE BEFORE STARTING AT THE GYM

I am a language teacher and personal trainer living in the province of Almería, although at that time I worked in the agricultural sector. At the age of 25, I had never set foot in a gym, nor did I know what it was. I weighed over 100 kg and, of course, I was out of shape. I didn't understand why people went to the gym, and I thought they were all vain. I didn't even like those people and didn't understand that lifestyle. Back then, I smoked a lot and couldn't run more than 100 meters without getting winded, but I thought it was normal, since in the environment I moved in, everyone was more or less like me. Sports had never knocked on my door, I don't know if due to coincidence or simply because I avoided them.

Now I am 50 years old (my goodness), and after 25 years of experience in fitness and combat sports, with everyone's permission, I am going to dare to write a few lines describing all my experiences about all the myths and legends I have seen and heard in this world. Although I now have my own gym, for many years I enjoyed the "flora and fauna" of many gyms where I experienced the strangest things any gym-goer could imagine. Over the years, I have observed how humans deceive themselves to avoid feeling bad about themselves, and how they choose to hear only what benefits them. I have also seen how gym users spread rumors and false information among themselves, creating a paranormal mythology of training and sports nutrition to unimaginable levels, which have become entrenched over time, making it almost impossible to make people see that it isn't true, or that it doesn't work that way. In this book, I am going to try to demystify all those myths and legends of the fascinating world of fitness.

CHAPTER 2

I DON'T WANT TO GET TOO MUSCULAR

I have been trying to get huge for 25 years, trying to grow, giving everything to gain one more gram of muscle, giving myself the effort in each of the repetitions, in each of the series, in each training, each day, each week, each month, every year, and you hear someone say that they wouldn't want to get too strong. At that moment, you don't know how to react, if it weren't for the fact that you know that that comment comes from ignorance and without any type of malice. There are even women who don't want to work with weight, because they think they are going to wake up the next day with huge shoulders. Nothing is further from reality. Many people think that getting huge is an individual's choice. Getting a single gram of clean muscle takes a lot of work and discipline, daily perseverance and a lot of sacrifice. I believe that this is the only sport in which you can hear such idiocy. Nobody signs up for a tennis academy and explains to the teacher that they don't want to play like Nadal, or like Federer, and nobody signs up for a basketball academy and tells the teacher that they don't need to play like Michel Jordán, who is content with make the free throws. Obviously, they would take him for a fool. Well, in fitness, it does happen. People, beginners obviously, think and assume that it is a personal choice to have the body of Ronnie Coleman or Arnold Schwarzenegger. As I said before, that wouldn't happen in other sports. Muscle growth entails a discipline that is not seen in any other sport, since the bodybuilder is a bodybuilder 24 hours a day, 365 days a year. In this book I am going to mention the word bodybuilder many times, and by that I am not going to refer to the professional bodybuilder who competes on stage, but to any person who worships their body in order to reach their peak. high, both aesthetically and from a health point of view, so, from now on, I am going to use the word bodybuilder, to anyone who aims at muscle growth, whether for competitive purposes or not. There are many people who also think that competitive bodybuilders have such perfect bodies because they use doping substances. It is true that steroids make the path to reaching that goal much easier, but it is not everything. Nobody gets strong by injecting insulin, growth hormone or testosterone and lying on the couch. There is a lot of work behind this "unhealthy" supplementation. Professional bodybuilding, whether doping or not, requires a sacrifice that we could rarely find in any other sport.

The nonsense is such that there are people who don't want to train very hard, because they think they could get huge even if they didn't want to, as I said, that wouldn't happen in any other sport. Bodybuilding has always had many detractors, and I believe it is due to envy and ignorance of this noble sport. Nowadays there are still many young people who go to a gym for the first time, and if they see a photo on the wall of a professional bodybuilder, the first thing they say to the gym monitor is, "I want to get big, but I don't that much". Let's imagine that a mother encourages her child to play soccer, and on the first day she tells the monitor, "I want my child to learn to play, but not like Messi." I prefer not to say what the monitor would think at that moment.

On the other hand, there is the great degree of disrespect that a large number of people show towards athletes who want to take care of themselves and have a good physical appearance. We are always treated as conceited, self-centred and more. There is always the typical comment that we are obsessed with our body, but no one would ever say that Rafa Nadal is obsessed with the racket or that Miguel Indurain is obsessed with the bicycle. Why if it happens with the bodybuilder? Logically, here is the envy factor. Behind those words, like "that makes me sick" and similar nonsense, a level of envy and frustration is hidden when they are not capable of having the capacity for sacrifice that fitness athletes have.

I don't know how many hours a footballer, tennis player, or even a rugby player trains, but I imagine no more than 15 hours a week. A bodybuilder trains 24 hours a day. The bodybuilder goes to the movies and does not drink Coca-Cola or eat popcorn, he does not watch football while eating pizza and drinking beer, and even sometimes, when he goes to a wedding, he has to bring a Tupperware to eat his own food, and how does he reward all that effort? "They're all pimps who are obsessed."

Another thing that never ceases to surprise me is how people think they understand a lot about this topic. That is to say, when a person does not know anything about mechanics, he would never contradict a mechanic, when a person does not know anything about aeronautical engineering, he would never give his opinion on it, when a person does not know anything about medicine, he does not usually contradict a doctor, and when a person does not know anything about electricity, he would never contradict an electrician. However, here on the topic of bodybuilding and sports nutrition everyone thinks they know and it doesn't matter who the person is, it doesn't matter who the specialist is. A person, by the simple fact of having been to a gym for two or three months, is already qualified to contradict any professional in the sector. Everyone thinks they know a lot about muscle exercise, routines, nutrition, etc., and they dare, without having done sports in their life, to contradict people who are professionals in the sector. This would not happen in any other area of life; it would never happen in another sector.

CHAPTER 3

DO A LOT OF ABS TO LOSE FAT

There are thousands of myths and legends in the world of irons, but this is perhaps one of the most deep-rooted. There has always been a lot of talk that doing abdominal exercises can burn fat located in the abdomen, and the worst thing is that it continues to be said. Many celebrities who appear to be in good physical condition do a disservice to society by saying that they have that "chocolate bar" due to the countless abdominal exercises they perform, when they may not even do these types of exercises. This only adds more confusion to this type of myth, which, instead of trying to clarify it, we increase its legend even more. Some of these famous people claim to do

2,000 or 3,000 sit-ups a day, with the sole purpose of laughing at people, since they know that many people will believe them, and that they will get Cristiano Ronaldo's chocolate bar, by doing the same.

Nowadays it is well known that it does not work that way. It is impossible to burn localized fat from any part of the body. The body "burns fat" globally, without anyone being able to choose which part they want to burn that fat from. In fact, the last place where men usually lose fat is in the abdomen and women in the hips.

Let's clarify a little the idea of how fat is burned. There are three nutritional states; caloric surplus, normo-calorie and caloric deficit and unfortunately you can only be in a nutritional state. The caloric surplus is when more calories are ingested than are expended, the norm of calories is when the same calories are ingested as are expended, and the caloric deficit is when fewer calories are ingested than are expended.

For our body to use accumulated fat as fuel, it is necessary to ingest fewer calories than our body uses. That is, we need to be in a caloric deficit. Let's try to explain this a little better.

I eat 2000 calories, but with my daily physical activity I only use 1800. In this case I would have a surplus of 200 calories, which my body would store as fat (or muscle, if things are done right). Either way, those 200 extra calories would make me gain weight in 100% of cases.

On the other hand, there is the normal calorie. I eat 2000 calories, but my daily caloric expenditure is 2000 calories, which means I neither gain nor lose weight. I stay the same.

And now let's get to the interesting part of this topic.

if I eat 2000 calories, but my daily caloric expenditure is 2200, the 200 calories that are missing my body is going to take from the fat that I have accumulated, and that is what we commonly call "burning fat."

Unfortunately, there is no other way other than that. We can do all the abdominal exercises or any type we want, if there is no deficit, there is no weight loss. The more exercise we do, the more calories we will burn and the more likely we are to reach that deficit, but I insist, we must reach it, if not, there is nothing. Normally the exercise that will help us achieve this caloric deficit will be cardio vascular exercise or weight training, but in no case abdominal exercises.

So, abdominal exercises are useless? At no time have I said that. Abdominal exercises have a function, but it will never be fat loss. People in the world of irons, people who work with loads, must have a good abdominal belt to avoid hernias and other types of injuries. When we do abdominal exercises, we are strengthening that part of the body. It is scientifically proven that no matter how much abdominal exercise you do, it is very difficult for that muscle to grow. The abdominal muscle is a muscle that is already genetically given. So, what happens is that little will change because we work with this type of exercises, but what we can achieve is to have a lot of strength in that part of the body to avoid injuries, but our abdominal aesthetics will never, never, never change by doing that type of exercise.

CHAPTER 4

LONG SERIES TO DEFINE AND SHORT SERIES TO BUILDER MUSCLE

Here we find another myth that may not be as famous as that of abdominal exercises to lose belly but that is not far behind and that is when we say that to define you have to do long series and that to gain muscle mass you have to do short series. Nothing more far from reality. That, of course, is not the case, because the definition or gain of muscle mass will be determined by the nutritional state we are in, as we have explained in another chapter. There are three nutritional states, on the one hand, there was the caloric deficit, on the other hand, there is the calorie norm and on the other hand, there is the caloric surplus. It will depend on whether we are in definition or if we are in volume, but it will never depend on the fact that the series have more repetitions or fewer repetitions. On the one hand, there is the stimulus that is given to the muscle, which is what we get when we do an exercise and then the diet will determine where we are going, if we are going to do a definition or if we are going towards a volume, but it never does. It will determine the way we train. One thing is that when we are in definition there comes a moment, there comes a point in which the strength is diminishing and there comes a moment in which it is difficult for us to move heavy weights and we run the risk of injury and then sometimes we choose to lower a little weights and make longer series, but that as a consequence of the state of the definition in which we are, but not looking for the state of definition in that way. That's not the way. It is your body that will decide that you can no longer handle more kilos and that it will choose to do more repetitions. It is also not advisable to work with little weight, because according to the latest studies, if we do not train hard, if we do not train very heavy, when we are in definition, there is a greater risk of losing muscle mass, which is not a very good idea either, but it is true , that there comes a time when you have to lower the weight, but that does not mean that you have to do it at the moment in which we are going to start a definition and that to burn more fat you have to do more repetitions. That doesn't work like that, because as we have said before, that will only be dictated by the nutritional status in which we find ourselves. I believe that this whole myth is given, this legend is given because people think or have the feeling that the more repetitions they do, the more cardiovascular exercise they are doing and that they are burning more calories, and that is not the case. This is not the case, because a very heavy series, with many and many kilos, can make your heart work harder than with a long series, that is, you do not have to be burning more calories with more repetitions than with a few. repetitions. I think that's where the myth comes from, but in any case, the nutritional status will tell where we are going and not the number of repetitions.

When this type of comment comes from the typical gym user, who has been in a gym for three months, and who already forms his own opinion about it based on the things he has heard, and in this case, it would not be very important. The problem comes when this comment comes from the shift monitor who is in the room working. That does a lot of damage. It hurts the staff a lot because people believe in that monitor. I have heard these comments about long series to define and short series for a volume. I've even heard it from the gym owner. Eh, then of course, since then you are not going to hear it from normal and ordinary people. People think that if the gym owner says it, he will know more than me. Of course, sometimes ignorance in these types of topics is not only in the public or in the client who goes to the gym, sometimes it is even in the professionals, and that is a big problem. I remember very well, a long time ago, a great friend of mine who lives in Germany, Javier Sanz, although he is better known for "El Barraco aus Frankfurt am Main". Well, he lived in Germany, now he lives in Switzerland, and he even told me the following. Within the same training, do both things at the same time. Series for volume and series to define. I think he was telling me something like that. "Alfredo, I have done a high series workout to define and then I have done a few short series to gain volume and so in the same workout I give volume and definition to the muscle." Of course, as if that depended on it, on the number of repetitions, and that is not the case, because as we repeat again and, in this book, I am going to repeat it many times, that does not depend on the exercise, that depends on the nutritional status in whichever we are, and of course, unfortunately we only have one mouth and one digestive system, and we cannot be in different nutritional states at the same time. If we are in definition, we are in definition, and if we are in volume, we are in volume. Well, this peculiar character, and great friend, also told me a very curious thing, and that is that he did not like to train his legs, because when his legs grew a lot, it gave the impression that his penis was smaller. That said, quite a character.

When we do the exercise, we give a stimulus to the muscle and depending on the nutritional state we will go one way or another.

CHAPTER 5
CARBOHYDRATES AT NIGHT MAKE YOU FAT

Here are some of the best-known myths in history. Who hasn't heard of this myth? I believe that the question should not only be that, but what is more, who does not share this myth? This myth should be one among many, but nevertheless it is one of the most important, not only because of the number of followers it has, but because it is a myth that after many years of existence, is still alive in our society, not only because of a large population that is "ignorant on the subject", but what is even worse, even some medical professionals, who do not retrain, and who also continue to say it, with the great damage that a comment like this causes. to society.

Many people even dare to put a time on "this evil eating of food." Some say that from 5 in the afternoon, others a little later, around 7, and others only move it to dinner. Incredible as it may seem, I see few people on television trying to deny such stupidity. I wouldn't dare say what percentage of the population believes in this myth, but possibly more than 80%.

Now let's see the origin of this fascinating myth. Many people think that the body's metabolism slows down after a certain time of day to facilitate rest, that is, to make it easier to fall asleep, which is true. So where is the myth? The problem is that this slowing down of metabolism is so insignificant that it practically does not affect the fact that this carbohydrate intake makes us gain weight. Once again, we must remember that what makes us gain weight is the calorie surplus, and that it does not matter at all what time of day we eat food. Calories are equally fattening at any time of the day. Let's also take the opportunity to mention the famous myth that breakfast is the most important meal of the day, and in which we "turn blue to eat crap", without any remorse, since at that time food does not make you fat. Well, once again, and nothing could be further from the truth, it is another nonsense, since breakfast is the most unnecessary meal of the day, since after having slept 8 hours, what the body least needs is for us to give it food, since after so many hours of inactivity, you do not need to recharge any energy, quite the opposite.

But how has this myth managed to penetrate society so deeply? Well, the truth is that I don't know, but the truth is that this myth is a classic among the classics, and so strongly rooted that it is almost impossible to try to convince the majority of society about its falsehood. These are things that we pass on from one to another and after many years and through many generations, it is almost impossible to deny, even as I have mentioned before, among the medical class.

The famous comment about how harmful it is to eat carbohydrates at night can be heard everywhere, from television series, news programs, radio programs, and what is worse, even in sports environments, where this already had to be more than demystified.

CHAPTER 6

I DON'T GROW DESPITE TRAINING VERY HARD

Once again, we are faced with another classic from our environment. Many people claim that they do not get the results they deserve despite the hellish work they do in the gym. Well, nothing could be further from the truth. The vast majority of these people do not work hard enough.

It is well known that human beings are very subjective with themselves. Normally we have the perception that we deserve more than what we get. We always think that we eat little for what we gain weight, and that we get few results for what we work for.

It is true that there are many people who go to the gym daily and spend a lot of time there, but that is not synonymous with working hard. We all know the typical gym user, who has been there for 20 years, and who still has the same body he had the day he started going. Normally these types of people attribute this problem to genetics, or failing that, to the fact that they are "natural athletes", who, since they do not use doping, cannot achieve the improvements that others achieve.

We must make one thing very clear, hard work is not a function of the hours we spend in a sports centre, but rather the muscle congestion we reach there.

Let's take the example of "Pepe". Pepe is a "great athlete who goes to the gym 4 times a week." Pepe goes to the gym every day at 6 pm, after a hard day at work. When he arrives at the gym, he goes to the locker room, changes his clothes while chatting with his colleagues about how his day went, or about the soccer game the night before, without rushing, since his work day has ended and he is to the gym to relax. After half an hour of talking, he heads to the weight room, very well equipped and full of energy, ready to face a long, hard and exhausting weight training session.

Once there, let's not forget that it is already 6:30 p.m., he greets all the acquaintances he meets, chats a little with each of them, with some he even comments on the challenging training session he is about to attend. to confront. He takes a general look around the room, notices that there are some very pretty girls in the cardio area, and without thinking twice he decides that he is going to start warming up a little in said area, using the elliptical bike next to some of those girls. so attractive Pepe dares to start a small conversation with one of them, while the warm-up begins, of course at a speed that does not prevent him from having a normal conversation with the girl, and 20 minutes later he decides that the time has come to face that infernal training you have in mind.

It's already 6:50 p.m. He takes another general look around the room, to see which machine is free, since he doesn't care what exercise he is going to do, since he doesn't give it the greatest importance either. In the distance he sees a free femoral curl machine, to which he quickly and quickly goes, just in case someone arrives before him. He spreads his towel over it and he already knows that this machine is his, that no one can take it away from him. Very calmly, he takes another look around the room, when surprisingly he sees an acquaintance whom he greets without hesitation, and after 10 minutes of chatting, it is already 7:00 p.m., his friend asks him if he can share a machine with him, which he accepts without hesitation. They exchange series, while they chat with each other, and show each other some Facebook or WhatsApp videos. Of course, they both do the exercise with the same weight, so they don't have to change the weight, and half an hour later the exercise is finished.

It's already 7:30 p.m. Pepe takes another general look around the room, when he notices that there is a shoulder press machine, which is empty. Limping and half-limping, due to the brutal exercises he has just performed on the hamstring curl machine, he heads to said machine. He spreads his towel again, clean and well scented, since Pepe has not yet broken a sweat (nor is it his goal, by the way) when he notices the presence of another great friend. They greet each other and he tells him a little about the wild training he is doing, and since they are very close friends, Pepe offers him to share a machine with him, which he accepts without hesitation, since his friend does not have a training plan with a goal too clear. After 20 minutes of hellish training, they say goodbye and Pepe looks up again.

It's already 7:50 p.m., almost two hours into a brutal workout, when in the free weights area, he sees an empty bench. Pepe spreads his towel again, and realizes that he has forgotten his water bottle at home. Since such a hard workout causes a lot of thirst, he does not hesitate to go to the water dispenser to buy a bottle, but of course, he has left the money in the locker of the locker room where he has to go first. Along the way he greets friends and acquaintances with whom he exchanges a few words. She buys the bottle of water and returns to the bench. Logically, 15 minutes have already passed, which means it is 8:05 p.m. He places the bar on the bench, some plates and prepares to do some sets, with light weight of course, because he is afraid of getting injured and does not want his fascinating sports career to be cut short by overdoing it in training. It seems that Pepe has also heard about overtraining, which is why he takes special care not to limit himself too much. Between series Pepe has received some messages on his mobile phone, which he has not hesitated to read and respond to very politely. After 3 sets of bench press, Pepe touches his chest a little, as if he had it very congested, a Ronnie Coleman style after doing 15 repetitions with 350 kilos.

20 minutes after those very hard series, it is already 8:25 p.m., Pepe decides that he wants to do a little cardiovascular exercise, since after that muscle destruction that he has just done to his body, he also thinks that it is good to burn a little fat. Sore and exhausted, Pepe heads to the cardio area, ready to finish off his sporting feat with a cardiovascular session that not even Arnold Schwarzenegger himself would have dared to do when he was younger. Pepe sees a treadmill which is free, and coincidentally next to the treadmill, there is an acquaintance. He gets on it, selects a speed that allows him to have a conversation with his friend next door, and after 35 minutes of a hellish marathon, only suitable for professional Kenyan marathoners, he concludes his very hard training and heads limping and badly injured to the locker room. where you are ready to take a shower. It's already 9:00 p.m.

Once showered and well cleaned, well perfumed with deodorant and cologne, he chats with his locker roommates about the training he has just completed. His colleagues congratulate him for such a tremendous feat and Pepe goes home, after making a great effort to get into the car, since such muscular work has left him practically incapable of carrying out any daily activity in life.

Pepe arrives home at 9:15 p.m., and tells his family that he has trained from 6:00 p.m. to 9:15 p.m. (the car ride also counts for him), that is, 3 and a quarter hour.

How many "Pepes" do we all know, right? Of course, when Pepe gets home, he opens the refrigerator and eats the first thing he finds, since he thinks that after that champion training that he just did, it doesn't matter what he eats, he will grow just the same. manner.

Well, from my humble point of view, this is the reason why we do not progress in the gym despite "TRAINING" more than 3 hours a day.

CHAPTER 7

GENETICS AND OBESITY

As we have already said in another chapter, human beings tend to convince themselves to do the right thing so as not to feel bad about themselves. Who has not heard the typical comment "I don't understand what's wrong with me, I don't eat anything and I gain weight."

Before I start demystifying this myth, I have to say that there are people who may have endocrine problems, thyroid problems, etc., and they would have nothing to do with everything I am going to write below. It must also be said that there are many people who say they have this problem, but here I have to say that there is only 0.001% of the world population with this type of problem, while there is a much larger percentage of people who are obese.

Well, I have bad news for all of you. No one gets fat from air. Throughout a life fully dedicated to fitness and sports nutrition, I have heard countless excuses of all kinds, to eat whatever we want and blame external factors for our extra kilos.

We always tend to think that we eat little and train a lot, when normally the opposite is true. More than one client has told me that his obesity is not because he eats too much, but because it is due to his genetics. That he has no choice but to be fat because in his family everyone is fat. Let's see, in a traditional family, the mother does the shopping for the house and is the one who cooks for the whole family. As a result of this factor, the entire family eats the same way, unless there is someone who wants to take care of themselves in a different way.

If in that family there is no culture of taking care of oneself, if one has never paid attention to what one eats, normally the food in that family is going to be a disaster, since the easiest thing is to eat junk food, because it is easy to prepare and affordable it is. We have this type of fast food everywhere and in the vast majority of cases it requires almost no preparation. Sometimes it's as simple as heating a pizza in the microwave.

If you are in a supermarket and you see someone who is overweight, you just have to look at their shopping cart to realize that they are not overweight due to a genetic factor. The issue of gaining weight is a matter of addition and subtraction. The more calorie surplus there is in the diet, the more weight we gain. Of course, it is easier to achieve that caloric surplus with a poor diet than by eating healthy. Each gram of carbohydrates has 4 kcal, as does each gram of protein, while each gram of fat has 9 kcal. Quickly assimilated carbohydrates, that is, sugars, are very easy to ingest and are the ones that the body can most easily store in adipocytes as a fat reserve. Although it is true that there are people more likely to gain weight, you have to eat the calories in order to gain weight. Imagine that we hire a bricklayer to build a house, but we do not provide him with bricks, sand or cement. Could you build the house? How can we gain weight if we do not give the body the necessary tools? Conclusion: Without a caloric surplus it is impossible to gain weight. You have to eat calories to gain weight. They don't float through the air until they reach you. You have to eat them first.

However, you can be thin for genetic reasons, but never the other way around. There are people with such a fast metabolism that their body "burns" everything they eat. These people are never in a caloric surplus because their body doesn't allow it. Everyone knows someone who eats a lot and we don't know where they put all that they eat. But the other way around is impossible. There are people who don't want to be so thin and go on special diets to gain weight and they can't. But the other way around is not possible, it is impossible. We need the extra calories to store them as fat.

CHAPTER 8

GAIN MUSCLE MASS AND LOSE FAT AT THE SAME TIME

This is also a classic among classics. Who hasn't heard it before. I wouldn't know what position to classify him into, but it's clear that it's something that all of us coaches have heard hundreds of times throughout our professional careers. Without a doubt, it is the dream of every beginner who goes to a gym for the first time. It is also called "body recomposition."

Unfortunately, this is a comment that is not only said by those who do not understand the subject, but also by some professionals who maliciously play with the enthusiasm of young kids who come to a gym for the first time. As we have already said in previous chapters, there are 3 different nutritional states. The caloric surplus, the normal calorie and the caloric deficit. Logically, we only have one mouth and one digestive system, so we can only be in one nutritional state at the same time.

To gain muscle mass you have to be in a caloric surplus and to burn fat you have to be in a caloric deficit. The body cannot gain muscle mass if it does not receive more calories than it burns and the body cannot burn fat if it does not burn more calories than it ingests.

So, what is the origin of this myth and why is it so well known? Apart from ignorance in this world of fitness, there is also the illusion that miracles happen. Many people completely believe that this can happen, and even claim that it has happened to them. It is true that there is one thing that can happen. When a person goes to the gym for the first time and has never worked their muscles, the following case may occur. Normally, they usually do so while they are somewhat overweight, so one of the first objectives that the monitor on duty focuses on (if he or she cares about it, of course) is to lose weight. The first thing is to lower that fat mass index, which apart from being quite unsightly, can also be harmful to your health.

At the same time that this fat is being "burned", and we are losing weight, there are muscles that have never worked before and that have begun to do so. As we removed that layer of fat that covers the muscles, we began to see muscles that we had never seen before, since they were buried under that layer of fat. At the same time, these muscles have begun to move and be active, so they may even be a little firmer and it may give us the sensation that they have grown, but as I just said, that is only a sensation, since If we have lost weight on the scale it is because we were in a caloric deficit, making it impossible for there to have been any growth in lean mass.

But of course, as we have already said in another chapter, it is very difficult, and I would say almost impossible, to try to convince people that this works like this, because as we have already mentioned previously, this is a sector in which everything the world thinks it is an expert.

So that miracle cannot happen under any circumstances. But now comes the icing on the cake. In itself, what we have just explained is impossible, but there are other people who claim that they do not lose weight, because despite being "burning" a lot of fat, at the same time they are gaining a lot of muscle, and that is the reason for the because the scale shows the same as the first day. This case is more spectacular than the previous one, because in the previous case, at least the individual was losing fat, without gaining any muscle, but at least he was losing fat, but in this last case, what the scale is telling us, is that this "athlete" is doing absolutely nothing.

If after being in the gym for 3 months the scale tells us that we weigh the same, this means that we have not done anything, based on what we have said previously, and you cannot be in 2 nutritional states at the same time. I couldn't tell you how many times I've heard this comment. I have even heard it from close friends, with whom, in order not to fully enter into a discussion, I prefer to leave the subject aside, since there would be no way in the world to make them see that this "miracle" of nature is impossible.

Anyone who understands a little about bodybuilding knows that there are two stages in this sport. On the one hand, there is the volume stage, in which athletes try to gain the maximum possible muscle mass, without being able to prevent some fat from also accumulating due to this caloric surplus, and on the other hand there is the definition stage. in which we try to get rid of that fat that we have achieved in the volume stage with the aim of being able to show off and show our muscles in the most expansive way possible. Professionals have to go through these two stages every year, however, newbies who go to a gym for the first time say they are able to do both things at the same time.

CHAPTER 9

QUIT SMOKING GET FAT

Although this is a myth of life itself, I also wanted to mention it in this book, since we also hear it a lot in gyms and I think it is worth commenting on.

Who doesn't know someone who has gained weight after quitting smoking? Everyone, right? This myth does not belong exclusively to the world of iron, but to life in general, which is why I was not sure whether to talk about it.

Smoking kills, and we all know that. I have smoked for over 30 years, which I am not very proud of. We start smoking because we want to pretend that we are adults and the only thing we are doing is killing ourselves while we are alive. Millions of people die every year from lung cancer and we continue to smoke. In fact, my father also died of lung cancer. Every time I see a 14-year-old smoking or vaping on the street, I don't know if I feel like crying or slapping him. My mother has always said that we should be old before being children so as not to commit the stupid things that are done in youth.

But hey, let's analyse a little the relationship between quitting smoking and gaining weight, which is the topic that concerns us now. Thousands of people claim that the simple act of quitting smoking causes them to gain weight. Nothing could be further from the truth, this is a falsehood.

You may be thinking that I am a pain in the ass when it comes to calorie surplus, but once again I feel obliged to mention it. "WITHOUT CALORIE SUPERAVIT IT IS IMPOSSIBLE TO GET FAT."

Without further ado, let's get to the heart of the matter. When we stop smoking, we enter a state of panic, nervousness, wanting to stop living, not finding meaning in life, etc. We think that life will not be the same without that cigarette. That coffee without a cigarette, that beer without smoking, that gathering without smoking with others, that cigarette after eating, etc. Of course, that emptiness has to be replaced with something, right? That's right, and how do we do it? Eating everything that comes our way, even things we didn't even eat before, but it doesn't matter, we have to fill that void.

If in our smoking stage we ingested 2000 kcal, now that we have just stopped smoking, we start ingesting 2500 or 3000. What is going to happen to us? We all know the answer, that, due to this increase in calories, logically we are going to gain weight. But what would happen if we didn't increase our caloric intake? Indeed, we would not gain weight. What makes you fat is not quitting smoking, but rather the increase in calories that we eat to try to appease a nervousness that will continue, because the only thing that excess calories will produce is more stress, since from that point onwards moment we are going to have two problems instead of one, that the nervousness of the lack of nicotine will be joined by the depression of seeing that we are gaining weight.

Many doctors recommend going on a diet before quitting smoking, not for nothing, but because they already know that the ex-smoker will pay for his nervousness by eating more than he should.

I think it is not worth expanding further on this myth, since I think it has become clear (I hope for most people), and that there is nothing hormonal or paranormal in quitting smoking, but rather we try to counteract that nervousness. eating, and once again it must be said, that it is excess food that makes us gain weight.

CHAPTER 10

WATER BEFORE EATING LOSES LOSS

This is another pearl. Like all myths and legends, anyone tells a staunch follower of this "nonsense" that this is not true.

In this chapter we are not going to go into much detail, since its simplicity is not enough. There are people who also say that drinking water before eating makes you lose weight and that after eating you gain weight. Of course, I would like someone to explain it to me, not for nothing, since the "nonsense" falls apart due to its weight, but to hear the explanation. I have always said that you can learn a lot from anyone. In fact, if I am writing this book, it is because of that, having listened to a large number of people, although I do not share in any way everything I have heard. That's why this book deals with "myths and legends", things that are nowhere near reality.

Water has no calories. What does that mean? Indeed, something that has no calories cannot make you fat. Because? Because if it does not have calories, it cannot help overcome or achieve the caloric surplus necessary to gain weight.

Ok, now let's demystify the myth. If we drink a certain amount of water before eating, logically that water will occupy a certain space in our stomach that will prevent us from eating other types of food. That is to say, if we normally ingest an amount of 2000 kcal, without drinking water before starting to eat, and now we drink 2 litters of water before eating, it is evident that we are going to have difficulties in ingesting those 2000 kcal, not because nothing, but simply due to space issues. Therefore, it is possible that we ingest only 1500. In that case, of course we are going to lose weight, since we are going to reduce the number of calories we were ingesting. But what would happen if, despite drinking 2 litters of water, we still eat the same amount of food? Do I really have to explain it?

Well, in this case the number of kcal ingested would be the same, so we should not even consider that we were going to lose weight simply by drinking a lot of water.

The thing about drinking water after eating makes you fat, I'm not going to waste a second trying to demystify it, since I don't think you would even take me seriously.

CHAPTER 11

MY LEGS DON'T GROW

Well, here we all have to confess. Who works their legs correctly? Who strives to the point of exhaustion? Do we really give it our all when we train the lower body? Do you really want me to tell you the answer?

Okay, I don't think it's necessary. Correct leg training involves hellish overexertion. We are all used to seeing people with super muscular upper bodies but who leave a lot to be desired in their lower bodies. Because?

Working the lower body requires a huge effort. Our legs work daily, even if we don't like sports. Everyone has to walk, so they are muscles used to daily work.

When we train legs, we recruit many muscle fibres and the cardiovascular demand is immense. The famous squats, lunges and press are the most feared exercises for most mortals.

Thousands and thousands of gym users train their entire body muscles, but leave the lower body aside. The excuses are numerous. Since I don't need it since I play soccer every Thursday or I don't see it necessary since I never wear shorts. I don't want to leave aside those who claim that they don't train legs because they grow too much and then they don't fit in any pants. I have yet to see any bodybuilder walking around in their underwear on the street. Logically, the truth is different. Apart from the great effort involved in leg training, then comes the day or days later.

When we train a muscle and the following days we feel sore, just try not to use those muscles (as much as possible) to avoid pain. And, what happens with the legs? Well, we have no choice but to have to walk. We cannot avoid this exercise that we have to do daily. There are countless problems that arise when we have sore legs. Sometimes it is difficult for us to walk, climb a staircase, sit or get up from a chair, get into a car, bend over, get up from the toilet, get out of bed, etc., etc.

So, to avoid all this, we invent thousands of excuses to avoid having these painful and uncomfortable sensations.

Here we also have to mention the great importance of working these muscles. Many of the few people who dare to train their legs do so gently, with machine quadriceps extensions, femoral curls and other less stressful exercises than the dreaded squats. Leg training not only benefits them, but the rest of the body. The hormonal influence of leg training benefits the rest of the body. Arnold already said it, "if you want your biceps to grow, do squats."

In conclusion, the legs do not usually grow in the vast majority of people who go to the gym because they do not train them with sufficient intensity. It is well known that they are more complicated muscles to grow, but if we add to this the terrible fear, we have of soreness the next day, then we make an odyssey about training them, and we come to the conclusion that I have a genetic problem with them, when the only thing we have is a problem of lack of effort with their training.

CHAPTER 12

THE NUTRITIONIST, THAT MYTHOLOGICAL BEING

In this chapter we are going to make a special mention of the nutritionist. That mythological, strange and at the same time picturesque being, who has more than earned the sky, seeing everything he has to "deal with" every day.

The nutritionist is a character that I admire, as it could not be otherwise, since I am also an expert in sports nutrition. He is a very unique professional, since he is someone, we usually hire his services to tell us what we already know (as long as the goal is to lose weight), but with the aggravating factor that we do not pay attention to him and are not happy. With this, we also criticize it when the objectives do not reach.

Everyone knows someone who has been to more than 3 or 4 different nutritionists, with the goal of losing weight, and coincidentally none of them have found the key to reaching that goal. . What a bad luck! The nutritionist usually has 2 objectives. The first of them is usually to help lose weight, and the second and no less important, is not to lose the client. Without a doubt, the second objective is much more difficult than the first, since the first is simply achieved with what was already mentioned in previous chapters, "calorie deficit."

Not losing the client is not an easy task. It must be taken into account that the nutritionist is working with people, with feelings and in many cases, with people who do not have much willpower when it comes to facing healthy eating habits. It is at that moment when this professional has to "grant" his client some whim or another. When a patient arrives for the first time at a nutritionist's office, he or she does a short interview inquiring about his or her eating habits and also learns what foods are the most difficult for them to do without. There are people who often say that they cannot eat without bread, well, those people are recommended to take 200 grams of bread at each meal. There are others who cannot do without ham, because the nutritionist recommends that they eat ham on their morning toast. Others have a weakness for chocolate, as they are also given a little license so that life does not become bitter and they can enjoy this succulent delicacy.

Well, so far so good. The problem worsens when three people, who follow the wise advice of different professionals, get together to chat, and tell each other what their nutritionist authorizes them to eat. Of course, now we begin to listen and draw the conclusions that best suit us when it comes to satisfying our palate without any regrets. One tells the other two that his nutritionist lets him eat bread, the other that his nutritionist lets him eat ham, and the third that his nutritionist lets him eat chocolate. What conclusion do the three subjects reach? Because bread, ham and chocolate don't make you fat. Of course, the nutrition expert has never said that. He has only given each of his clients the whim of satisfying their palate a little with the desire to make life a little easier for the patient and not lose that client, but knowing that this small gastronomic license was not the best choice. for the patient's goals.

Another problem that we usually face when it comes to nutrition problems is constant customer deception. When we are following a strict nutritional plan in which the patient should have lost 2 kg in a month and he comes to you saying that he has gained two kilos, but the reason is not explained, since he has followed the diet to the letter. Well, very well, we must tell all those people that two plus two equals four, and that, although the numbers are not round, they are not square either.

There are other people who not only deceive the nutritionist, but also everyone around him. There are those who, when they go to eat at a restaurant with other people, barely eat anything, and everything they eat is very healthy, and, due to their appearance, you don't have to be very intelligent or an expert in nutrition to know that this food is not what they eat daily. I call that self-deception, because the rest are not being deceived.

When a nutritionist sends a nutritional plan to his client, in 99% of cases it should work. But of course, you have to do what it says on paper. what is the problem? There are people who spend their entire lives jumping from one nutritionist to another in search of that miracle. Looking for that nutritionist who can make them lose weight by eating what they want and of course, that's where the problem comes, since that doesn't exist. That is to say, there are people who go to a nutritionist and do not lose weight, logically because he does not pay the slightest attention to them. He goes to another one, he doesn't lose weight either and of course, he is looking for someone who will make him lose weight by eating whatever he wants, pizza, beer, industrial pastries. etc... There are people who spend their entire lives jumping from one nutritionist to another and all his life in a state of obesity, since he does not lose weight. He doesn't lose weight because he doesn't pay attention to anyone, but any nutritionist can make anyone lose weight, not for nothing, but because it is tremendously easy.

On the other hand, there is the nutritionist's mischief. There are nutritionists who, knowing that the food they are sending to their client is not the most appropriate to achieve their goal, as we have already mentioned before, have to cheat a little and send something so that the client is happy, because if a nutritionist is very harsh with his client and that client hears from other nutritionists that he allows his clients to eat ham or eat pizza or drink beer, they are going to abandon him and go in search of the other, so sometimes, knowing that what they are sending is not the most correct thing, they have to do it.

CHAPTER 13

OVERTRAINING

This myth that we are going to talk about now may not be as deeply rooted in society as others, but that does not mean it is unimportant, and it is about overtraining. That state that many people say they reach due to the stratospheric training they do that prevents their progress. My personal trainer has always said that overtraining does not exist, that the state of fatigue that we can occasionally reach is due to "undernutrition and lack of rest."

Those who advocate the existence of this evil claim that they have the key to not reaching this unfortunate state of deterioration, and that it consists of training less. Those of us who have enjoyed the "flora and fauna" of gyms for decades know that this is not true. As I already presented to you in chapter 6 titled "I DO NOT GROW DESPITE TRAINING VERY HARD", to our friend "Pepe", I believe that someone similar to Pepe, or at least with the same desire to train as him, was the one who invented This thing about overtraining. In the fitness world there has always been a rumour that you had to do 9 sets for small muscles, and 12 sets for large muscles. Well, scientific and practical evidence has shown us that this is not the case. It is true. With this type of training, we do not give our body enough stimulus to make it grow, so we are not going to overtrain it by any means.

Before talking a little more about overtraining, let's explain how and why muscles grow. When we are in the gym and train "hard", we are subjecting our body to both physical and mental stress. After a long and hard training session we suffer many micro muscle tears, which our body wants to repair later. For this repair to take place, sufficient rest and the appropriate amount of nutrients are necessary. If all this is carried out, there will be a muscular adaptation to the suffering that our body received with the exercise, repairing itself and becoming stronger, so that the same thing does not happen to us again in the next weight training session. But of course, since we want to grow, what we are going to do in the next session is increase the intensity of the training in order to be able to cause muscle damage again and for this cycle of muscle destruction and repair to take place. That way, we will grow muscularly.

As we mentioned in the previous paragraph, training must be hard for the adaptations we are looking for to occur, otherwise all the work will have been in vain. The majority of people who do not progress in the gym are not because of the dreaded overtraining, but rather because they are lazy. To reach that so-called state of overtraining, I don't know how many sets I would have to do, but I'm sure it must be a lot, since there are those who work for hours in the gym, and quite hard, and have never experienced that state. So, don't be afraid to do more than 9 sets, you are not going to overtrain, quite the opposite, your body is not going to notice and we will be wasting time.

In short, I think we should forget about that word that does so much damage to this noble and sacrificial sport, train hard and leave laziness at home when we go to the gym.

CHAPTER 14

PROTEIN SHAKES VS STEROIDS

This is one of the myths that bothers me the most, when we confuse natural supplementation with anabolic steroids. It bothers me not only because normal people are confused but because even professionals in the sector and what is worse, medical professionals also do it.

Many people demonize everything that has to do with bodybuilders and gyms, even going so far as to put egg whites in the same bag. I remember one time, more than 20 years ago, I was in a gym and a kid of about 18 was about to drink a protein shake in the locker room after his training session. At that moment the room manager appeared and told him that this was prohibited in that gym. The young customer was trying to explain to him that what he was going to drink was a simple whey protein shake and that this was not bad for his health. At that moment, the monitor on duty, seeing that the client was not obeying him, ran to look for the gym director. They both started yelling at the young man, telling him that his liver was going to burst if he took that, and that he was going to be expelled from the sports centre. Well, unfortunately those are the professionals we have. I can understand that some older doctors who have not been trained much in these topics may have this type of confusion, but not in two young professionals who have just finished their degree at INEF (national institute of physical education), now called CAFYD (Degree in physical activity and sports sciences).

On many occasions I have a lot of doubt about the level of the Spanish university and the degree of preparation with which the students leave it. The truth is that I don't know what they study in that degree, when they don't know how to differentiate between legal sports supplementation and doping.

Now let's see the pros and cons of sports supplementation. All products for sale in any supplement store are healthy and legal. All of them have passed rigorous safety checks and all of them are safe for health. In fact, the famous protein shake is made with whey, so it couldn't be healthier. As well as the rest of the supplements, creatine, branched chain amino acids, L-Carnitine, glutamine, etc. Let's say these would be the pros of legal sports supplementation.

Now let's see the cons. There is a big business around supplements. There are many bodybuilders whose source of income is the sale of these products. They try to make gym users believe that these types of products are miraculous and that they will achieve great results if they take this supplementation. Bodybuilding is a sport that is not very well paid, and its professionals have to resort to this type of business, although many of them are also personal trainers, just like yours truly.

The relationship between price and real results that these types of products offer us is very uneven. Although it is true that it can provide some benefit, around 5% of the final result, that is, almost nothing, the price is very high. So where is the catch? Bodybuilders who advertise these types of supplements, usually proteins, claim to have achieved the body they have thanks to these supplements, and that is not true. They have obtained it thanks to their great work, their great sacrifice and their great discipline with their diet, and of course, also with the help of other types of products that are neither healthy nor legal and which we will talk about below. Normally they come out with the bottle of protein in their hand and with a wardrobe that shows off their magnificent body, claiming that they have achieved it thanks to it, playing with the enthusiasm and economy of those young beginners who want and have the illusion of having a body like that of their idols, and from my point of view, that should be prohibited since it is "Fraudulent Advertising."

Everyone knows the existence of doping in the world of professional bodybuilding and in some cases in amateur bodybuilding as well, since there are many gym users who also consume this type of substance with the aim of maximizing their work in the gym. Anabolic steroids, whatever they are, growth hormone, testosterone, insulin, etc., are a great weapon to achieve those bodies that we see on television. Almost all the actors that we can see in the movies with super muscular bodies have used doping, since without these substances it is impossible to have muscle at that level. But like everything in life, this also has its contradictions, and the main one of all is that they are potentially dangerous to health. Many bodybuilders die within a year from the use of these substances, but most people do not realize since this is not a mass sport, and televisions do not a lot of echoes of it.

These types of substances are purchased on the black market, since they are illegal, and this increases their danger even more, since they have not passed a health control like legal sports supplements do. Steroids are dangerous even if you buy them at the pharmacy, so we can already imagine how dangerous they are when they come from the black market.

But, now, the fact that these substances are dangerous does not give people the right to treat bodybuilders the way they are treated. Bodybuilding is one of the most noble and sacrificial sports in the world, since the bodybuilder is a bodybuilder 24 hours a day, 365 days a year. It is a sport of personal improvement, in which you do not always compete with others, but with yourself. Some even carry a Tupperware when they have to go to a family member or friend's wedding. That is not done in any other sport. In the same way that these athletes have chosen to lead such a sacrificial life, they should also have the right to take the health risks they want, since it is their lives that are at stake and they should not be so criticized by others. of people.

Another thing that most people don't know is that simply taking a syringe and injecting any type of anabolic does not turn you into a superman overnight. Behind that syringe there is a huge job that very few people would be able to carry out. It is not about pricking yourself and lying on the couch waiting for your muscles to grow. Hormones help a lot with muscle development, but you have to work even harder than those who don't use them. Train hard, eat and rest, and so on every day of the year.

To summarize, it must be said that legal sports supplements are not dangerous, but they are not as effective as doping substances (not even close), and that even taking anabolic steroids you have to work a lot to build the desired body.

CHAPTER 15

WHEN YOU LEAVE FITNESS ALL YOUR MUSCLE WILL CONVERTE INTO FAT

Here comes another well-known myth. When you stop playing sports, all that muscle that you have gained over the years will turn into fat. "Another pearl that cannot be wasted." I don't get angry with this old saying, since it usually happens in a fairly high percentage of the population that when they stop playing sports, they get fat and lose muscle, but this doesn't happen directly as a consequence of it.

I explain. When a person practices fitness and takes care of their diet, it is most likely that they will be able to gain some muscle tone. We have all seen many footballers who are in great shape and when they retire or become coaches, they get fat. What is this natural phenomenon due to? Well, this doesn't have to happen if we do things right. When a person stops doing sports, they usually also stop taking care of their diet, and this is where the problem lies. When we stop playing sports, it is normal for our muscle tone to gradually decrease, but if we take care of our diet, even after stopping playing sports, we should not gain weight.

In previous chapters we have talked about the 3 nutritional states, calorie surplus, calorie norm and calorie deficit. When an athlete, professional or not, stops playing sports, his or her caloric expenditure also drops. When a footballer, cyclist, bodybuilder or tennis player stops playing sports and dedicates himself to something more sedentary, he no longer needs to eat the same number of calories that he did previously. If, in addition to not reducing the number of calories, we begin to give ourselves certain gastronomic indulgences that we did not indulge in before in our phase as athletes, what we are doing is increasing the number of calories, which will also come from a less healthy source and with a great capacity to increase our calorie surplus and with junk food that does not contribute anything good to our body.

If we combine the fact that we stop playing sports, and we start to lose muscle, with the fact that we start eating poorly, and we start to gain fat, our body composition changes, but in no case has our muscle become fat. We have lost muscle and gained fat, but they are totally different tissues.

Muscle has nothing to do with fat. A dog cannot become a cat, nor can a leg become a head. What happens here is that we are simultaneously changing our body composition. On the one hand, we are losing lean tissue with the cessation of sporting activity, and on the other hand we are gaining fat due to a poor diet, but in no case is one tissue being converted into another.

Sometimes we can also see that there are certain athletes who, despite having ceased their sporting activity, do not gain weight. This is because they have continued to eat in a healthy way and taking into account the number of calories. But this does not happen very often, since many of them, after many years of dietary restrictions, when they leave their profession, they are eager to try those whims that they could not allow themselves previously since they had to take care of their physical shape, and it is at that moment, when they start smoking, drinking and eating everything within their reach.

In conclusion, we have to say that muscle and fat are totally different tissues and that neither of them can be converted into the other, and that it only depends on us to change our body composition, that is, "muscle for fat.", instead of "muscle turning into fat."

CHAPTER 16
SWEATING BURNS FATT

Who doesn't know this old legend? And, what's more, it has been with us for so long that, would we be able to convince any of those who say this that this is not true? I think there is a better chance of a meteorite falling on us than of convincing them.

I remember, many years ago (but I think there are still those who do it), that many people went running at midday, when it is hottest, in summer, and wearing winter clothes, with the aim of sweating more and burning more. fat. Well, this doesn't work like that. Once again we have to resort to an expression that we have already used many times in this book, and it is the famous "calorie deficit."

Others are capable of spending hours in a sauna, with the same goal, to lose weight, and unfortunately that doesn't work either. After spending some time in a sauna, if we weigh ourselves, of course we have lost weight, but that weight we have lost does not come from fat, but from the water that we have eliminated by heat. The water that is lost due to excess heat, that is, through sweating, we will drink later. We do not lose fat by sweating, we only lose fluids, which we will replace later.

This sauna method is used by many athletes, including bodybuilders, when they have to give an estimated weight to be able to participate in a certain category of a championship. But they regain that weight once the weigh-in is over. They haven't lost any real weight.

There are people who even wrap plastic around their abdomen, with the aim of sweating that area, thinking that they are going to lose weight from that specific area. Well, nothing could be further from the truth, that doesn't work like that either. Fluids are lost, coming from all over the body, and which will be replaced later. We cannot ignore the danger of carrying out this type of activity, since heat stroke can have bad consequences for our health.

There are other people who turn to diuretics, natural and pharmacy. The result is the same, we are going to lose fluids which we will replace later. If we are competitors in bodybuilding or another sport in which we cannot exceed a certain weight, we will lose some weight momentarily, but in no case will we lose fat.

CHAPTER17

THE REBOUND EFFECT

-I'm on a diet.

- What do you say? Really? And how long does your diet last?

-It is a 3-month diet.

-Well, you'll see when the 3 months pass and you have the rebound effect.

I did not invent this conversation. It's real like life itself. The dreaded rebound effect, of which we must be alert in case it catches us treacherously.

Let's face it, I don't like the word "diet." That word that a priori seems normal, but that puts us in a state of alarm. I go on a diet when Christmas is over, or when Easter is over, or just before summer, or at the end of summer. And the well-known, "I start the diet on Monday", but that Monday never comes.

The word diet is for many like quitting smoking. It is a state that makes us nervous from minute one, it is a word that causes us chills, discomfort, bad mood, insomnia, depression, etc. I like diets that take time, as I mentioned in the conversation at the beginning of the chapter. "It's a 3-month diet." And the question is, what are you going to be when those 3 months pass? Do you have any plan, any project, is something paranormal going to happen? What is going to happen? Well, I'm telling you right now. In the hypothetical case that I last those 3 months, when that long-awaited day arrives, the day that my agony, my suffering, my torture ends, I am going to eat everything that comes my way. All the donuts I haven't eaten for 3 months, Coca-Cola with sugar, chocolate, cold cuts, pizza, ice cream, etcetera, etcetera.

Well, here I present to you the dreaded rebound effect. The rebound effect is nothing more than the nutritional change we make when we finish a diet. We've been on calorie restriction for a while, and now we're starting to "make up for lost time."

We went directly from ingesting 1500 calories for 3 months and went on to ingest 3500. A caloric surplus of 2000 calories that in three weeks means we gain 7 or 8 kilos on the scale. That's the rebound effect. This effect does not exist. It's only in our mind. It is the consequence of reversing a diet that we were doing in the best possible way to a true nutritional disaster. It is the effect of becoming like "Kiko" after a few months of abstinence from junk food.

I have said before that I don't like the word diet, since this should be a change of habits and not a 3- or 4-month diet. If we are in a state of overweight and we want to reverse it, we have to start eating well. For how long? Forever. What kind of diet? One that is sustainable over time, that helps us achieve our goals in a comfortable way, having our small nutritional whims, but being consistent that there are foods that must be eliminated from our daily lives. Being on a diet must be approached as a lifestyle change, instead of an ordeal.

If we are overweight and start a diet to lose weight progressively, when we reach our goal, we have to start with "plan 2". Plan 2 is to start with a normal calorie diet that allows us to remain in that state that we have reached, so that we neither gain nor lose weight. A diet that allows us certain gastronomic licenses, but without going overboard.

Nowadays, in the Western world we are lucky to have access to a wide variety of delicious foods that are not very high in calories. When we go to a supermarket, we find that practically everything we see has a light version. There are countless products that, despite being low in calories, have the same flavour as the original product. There are light soft drinks, smoothies, yogurts, flans, ice creams and many more. Many times, we think that there is a big difference in taste between the light product and the original, but in most cases, it is purely psychological. I could list countless cases that I have experienced with friends and family, who did not recognize which was the light product with the original. On the other hand, you also have to be careful with these light products that promise not to make you gain weight, but as I have said many times, if there is a caloric surplus, in the end we will gain weight, regardless of the product.

What happens is that by taking light products it is more difficult to achieve that surplus.

To conclude, I must say that the dreaded "REBOUND EFFECT" is caused by us. When the goal is reached, remember "plan 2", and the rebound effect will never catch us by surprise.

CHAPTER 18

I WILL START THE GYM AND DIET ON JANUARY 1

On the first of January. The most magical day of the year. The day when everything changes. We stopped smoking, we started playing sports, we started taking care of our diet, and of course, we signed up for an English academy. New Year's resolutions, or as they say in English, "New Year Resolutions".

If on December 28 we propose that on the 1st we are going to change our habits, both in sports and in our diet, then it would make sense, but when people say this on August 25, I think it is very far from reality. Millions of people start going to the gym on January 2, since it is closed on day one, and they go on a diet. 95% of them go to the gym until the 31st, because they have already paid for it, but they stop the diet on January 6th when we have to eat the famous "Rosco de Reyes". There are many gyms that live off January and June fees and we all know why. The month of January because it is the month of new challenges and the month of June because due to our ignorance, we think that we are going to get in shape to show off on the beach in just one month.

There are people who really change their habits in their lives that day, but usually that is not the case. When we need to look for a special day on the calendar to start doing something, it is usually not sustainable over time, and that is why we look for a day that gives us the motivation that we do not have.

If we are clear about it, we can start any Wednesday in the month of April, instead of a Monday. This strategy of starting a healthier life on the first day of the year is nothing more than an excuse to spend the whole year eating whatever we want, without any regrets, since we have convinced ourselves that we are going to start "that day." so strategic", even knowing that it is not true and that in a few weeks we will throw in the towel and we will consider it again for the following year, and so on year after year. It also happens a lot when someone goes to the nutritionist on a Wednesday, he gives them the diet, and he says, well, I'll start it on Monday. Why

Monday? And, what's more, what do you plan to do from today until Monday? We all know that, right? Indeed, devouring everything that comes our way, even things that we are not in the habit of eating, as if it were the last week of our life. With that aptitude it is difficult for us to change our habits. As I said in another previous chapter, we should not see the diet as an ordeal, counting the days we have been on and, worst of all, counting the days we have left to finish it, but rather a lifestyle change that will make it improves us.

Well, I think this chapter is going to be the shortest of all since I think this topic doesn't go any further. The only thing I would add is that any time is good to change habits, and not always leave it for that day, because we know that is not true. It is a false myth, a legend that does nothing but deceive ourselves.

CHAPTER 19

THE MUSCLE WHO HAS NO STRENGTH

This false myth is one of the ones that amuses me the most. It is unimaginable the large amount of nonsense that we are capable of saying out of pure envy. I have been hearing this false myth for many years and to this day we all continue to say it. How many times have we seen a group of kids training in a gym, (training is to call it that, let's say hanging out at the gym with friends), how they observe a well-muscled athlete who is doing an exercise with an impeccable technique, but according to them with very little weight, and here comes the typical comment: "So much muscle to lift that ....".

Many say them out of ignorance, and let's say that they could be forgiven, but most say it out of pure envy, because they would like to have that muscle mass, and they cannot, or do not have the spirit of sacrifice that must be had. to achieve it, and they console themselves by saying that those muscles are worthless, that they are the ones who are strong. Wow, they need to say that the more muscle you have, the more weakness there is.

I have heard it said by people who are new to the world of irons, but others are not so new, since they have been in the gym all their lives, but it is not noticeable, with a face and a tone of voice where the level of envy that those comments contain. When a friend tells you this, sometimes I have to keep quiet so as not to start an argument and make it seem like I want to pretend that I am the most expert in the world in the sector, but many times it is very difficult to digest these absurd words.

Well, now we are going to demystify this myth, and this absurd legend that does not make the slightest sense, from its origins. Where does all this come from? Why happens? Why does this seemingly strong man lift less than others who don't even look like they've ever played sports? GO FOR IT!

To perform a bodybuilding exercise correctly, we need to take several things into account:

- Good Technique, to minimize the possibility of injuries.

- Spirit of sacrifice, so that the muscle obtains the necessary stimulus.

- Correct intensity, both in the kilos we handle and in the rest times.

- Focus on exercise and disconnect from the environment.

- Leave the "EGO" at home, for me this last one is the most important of all.

When we are going to perform a bodybuilding exercise, our muscle needs the greatest congestion and the greatest possible isolation, to achieve the greatest results. This is normally achieved by doing the exercise very slowly, concentrating all our strength and our mind on those muscle fibres that we are destroying. Of course, when we do these movements so slowly, the amount of weight we can handle is less.

Let's put the first example in the barbell curl. A classic exercise for biceps growth. An exercise that should only involve your arms, right? To execute it, we should take the bar, place the elbows to the sides, hands supinated and flex the arms upward, bringing the bar to the neck as slowly as possible (concentric phase), and then slowly lower it towards the starting point (eccentric phase). This would be the correct execution of the exercise. Where is the problem? The problem is that, if we want to perform the exercise correctly, we will not be able to lift the same amount of weight as others who do not respect the technique. Many people, in the desire to lift more weight, pull the bar upwards, let it fall suddenly downwards, and do a lumbar hyperextension, that is, they throw their waist back, and some even jump to push themselves off, with the great risk of injury that this entails, and the uselessness of it, since we are working everything except the biceps.

It is at this moment where we begin to draw all the conclusions. Suppose there are two athletes in the same weight room who are performing this exercise. We are going to call them athlete "A", the one who does it with the proper technique, and athlete "B", the one who is working on the "EGO". "A" is performing it with 20 kg. Next to him is "B", doing it with 40. "B" is looking at "A" with signs of supremacy, very proud that he can handle more kilos than the muscular "A". If this athlete, whom we call "B", who is not doing anything at all, since that work is in vain, because his biceps are not even aware of it, since he is making all the effort with his lower back, had to do the same exercise with the technique that athlete "A" is using, he could not possibly carry more than 10 kilos, he would not even reach half the weight that athlete "A" is using. While, on the contrary, if we tell subject "A" that he forgets about technique, and lift everything he can, possibly he could handle 60 kg. Do we understand the difference now?

That muscular man goes to the gym to train his muscles and get results. He is not worried about the kilos he carries, but rather about working his muscles in the most efficient way possible and getting the most out of his training session. He also doesn't care about the weight that others carry since he doesn't even pay attention to them. If he did, he would break out into a smile. This is the reason why he has more muscles than those who are using more kilos, but in an inadequate way, because he is working correctly.

So, is the weight we lift important? Of course. The greater the weight we lift, the greater the results we will have "AS LONG AS WE RESPECT THE TECHNIQUE AND DO THE EXERCISE CORRECTLY", otherwise the training session will only have served two purposes. The first to make a fool of ourselves and the second to run the risk of injury.

If we are doing, for example, a bench press with 100 kilos, and we realize that we are not doing a complete movement due to the excess kilos, it is preferable to lower the weight and perform the entire exercise, since the exercise would be more effective. But of course, this does not matter to the conceited person who goes to the gym to boast that he lifts a lot of weight, because the only thing he is interested in is lifting more than others, and that is the reason why he lifts more kilos than the muscular person, surprising. , huh?

These types of people may have chosen the wrong sport. When we work on aesthetics, which is what fitness and competitive bodybuilding are all about, the important thing is muscle congestion, and not the amount of weight lifted. Muscle congestion does not have a direct and proportional relationship with the weight used. If what we want is to lift large amounts of weight, there are other disciplines for that, such as Weightlifting, Powerlifting or Strongman, etc.

After half a life in the world of fitness, as a gym user and as a personal trainer, I have been able to experience numerous experiences which may not seem credible. I remember one time, (by the way, I have also heard this experience that I am going to tell from my coach, so I have not been the only one who has experienced it), in a gym, a boy on a leg press, with more weight that this guy could move, he made such a small distance that he had not removed the safety of the machine, and he had not even realized it. We all know that, to perform this exercise correctly, we must bring our knees up to our chest and then stretch our entire legs. Well, we can imagine the movement that boy could do without removing the lock on the machine. This happens because when we want to do an exercise with more weight than we actually can, we have to shorten the movement, because otherwise it would be impossible, and that is the reason why, when we do exercises wanting to show others that we move a lot of weight, the risk of injury is monumental.

It also happens very often, when someone has just finished an exercise, before handing over the machine, the bench, etc., to another person, they ask, should I take the weight off? The person who is about to do the exercise quickly answers, "No, whatever, I do it with the same weight or more." If you watch him begin to do the exercise, you immediately realize that he cannot do it correctly, so he begins to do it with very poor technique, and when the person who gave him the machine leaves and is no longer present, this takes the opportunity to lose the kilos without the other person realizing it. The EGO can beat us!

Then we wonder why the muscular man has no strength. Well, it is very clear, he has twice the strength of the others, but he uses it correctly to get the most out of his exercises. There are other occasions in which the supposedly "strong guy", who has no strength at all, by the way, is about to do an exercise and asks for help from others with the excuse that he is doing it out of caution, as if caution were his thing. It worried him a lot. He lies down on a bench, ready to do some hellish sets of bench presses, with a friend on each side, and another behind. They help him remove the bar from the supports, because he can't even do that, and his friends begin to help him throughout the entire journey, both in the concentric and eccentric phases. Of course, he moos like a buffalo, and his companions tell him that they are not doing anything, that they are only accompanying him as a precaution, but that they are barely touching, and they are as red as tomatoes. These types of situations lead to many injuries and leaving the gym forever. I couldn't say what percentage of people leave the gym due to injury, but I could assure you that a large part of those who have been injured, they have been because they wanted to impress others by lifting more kilos than they really could.

To top it all off, there are those who, when they see someone stronger than them, claim that it is because they take doping substances, since they lift more kilos than them, and that they have less muscle. Of course, the problem is there, that we think that, for the simple fact of lifting more kilos, the muscles have to grow more. That could only be true, assuming that we are lifting more weight, but with the correct technique, since otherwise the exercise has been done in vain.

Well, I think this is going to be the last chapter. I don't know if this book I just wrote is a good book. I also don't know if it will be published and if it were published, I don't know if there will be anyone who likes it, but one thing is clear to me, I have done it with all the enthusiasm in the world with the intention of helping many people who are a little lost in this world that we sometimes complicate unnecessarily. Everything I have written, with more or less success, I have lived with my own experiences, without looking for any documentation anywhere and I hope you all liked it.